T0268198

The Simplest Alkaline Diet Guide for Beginners + 46 Easy Recipes

How to Cure Your Body, Lose Weight and Regain Your Life with Easy Alkaline Diet Cookbook

Eric P. Garvin

Contents

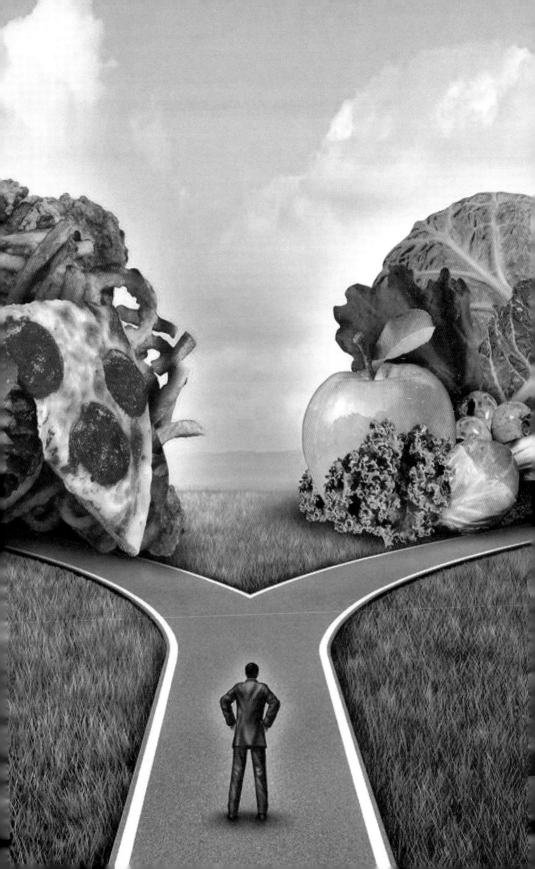

Introduction

Did you know that our blood pH must stay within a very small range, otherwise death or a serious illness can occur? Our bodies have a wonderful maintenance system to keep our blood in balance which is necessary for healthy human function. This system protects our blood, despite the circumstance, even at the cost of our own tissues. When our tissues become acidic, that in turn can result in improper function of some major systems, including; digestion, organ, repair from injury, and skin integrity.PH is really important to our bodies and there's a quick way to check if It's in balance and if it isn't there's also an easy way to fix it.

Our body's internal system requires a pH just over 7. We call this range; alkaline. (For example, dogs have an acid pH range that is on the lower end of the scale). Since we are human, our immunologic, enzymatic, and repair systems all function at their peak in this alkaline range. However, our metabolic processes - the processes of tissue repair, living, and food metabolism, produce a great deal of acid. To be able to maintain the alkaline state in our bodies, we need to be equipped with a few tools. These tools are all around us; water, oxygen, and acid-buffering minerals.

Examples

Exercise - When we exercise or use our muscles, we exert carbon dioxide and lactic acid. Lactic acid is by its nature acid and the carbon dioxide becomes acidic, turning into water, and carbonic acid.

Digestion–The digestion of a lot of foods comes with the acids. For example, phosphoric acid and sulfuric acid are produced by the metabolism of the sulfur and phosphorus found in many foods, such as beans, grains, and meats.

Immune Responses - Immune system reactions, such as hypersensitivities and allergies, indirectly and directly form large amounts of acidity.

Many environmental and lifestyle factors also contribute to the acid-alkaline balance. Let's look at stress as the first example; when we are under a great deal of stress, our acidity levels are likely to rise because of the demand on our cells to be more active. Constant hectic schedules, not enough sleep, and a poor or unbalanced diet can definitely add to this unhealthy condition.

Here's **the hard truth**… An underlying metabolic acidity (low pH) is a common and likely contributing factor to all autoimmune and deteriorative diseases.

Why? Because

An acid environment, for us humans, has several adverse **effects on cell metabolism** including

- Defective energy production
- Fluid edema and accumulation
- A possible increase in free radical production

What is the Alkaline Diet?

The alkaline diet is also known as the alkaline ash or acid-alkaline diet. It is based around the idea that the foods you eat can affect the alkalinity or acidity (the pH balance) in the body. Let me explain how this works; when you metabolize foods in the body and extract the calories/energy from them, you are actually burning the foods, except in a way that is controlled and slow. Burning the foods actually leave an excess of ash debris, just like when you burn wood in a furnace.

As it turns out, this ash can be acidic, neutral, or alkaline and enthusiasts of this diet, say that this ash can precisely alter the acidity of the body. So, eating foods that contain acidic ash **makes your body acidic** and if you eat foods that contain alkaline ash, it **makes your body alkaline**. Neutral ash has no effect. It's as simple as that.

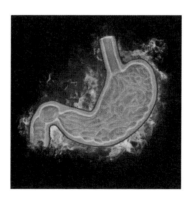

Acid ash is said to make you more vulnerable to disease and illness, however, alkaline ash is seen as protective. By replacing your acidic foods for more alkaline foods, you should be able to improve your health and "alkalize" your diet. Food items that leave an acidic ash include; phosphate, sulfur, and protein, while alkaline items include; potassium (1, 2), calcium, and magnesium.

Certain food groups are considered acidic, alkaline or neutral.

Acidic:

- Fish
- Meat
- Grains
- Poultry
- Alcohol
- Dairy
- Eggs

Neutral:

- Sugars
- Natural fats
- Starches

Alkaline:

- Legumes
- Fruits
- Vegetables
- Nuts

Meanings of each pH value

When studying the alkaline diet, it is important to understand the meanings of each pH value. Put simply, the pH value is the extent of how alkaline or acidic something is.

The pH value ranges from 0 to 14:

- (0-7) is acidic;
- (7) is neutral;
- **(7-14) is alkaline** (alkaline is also called basic).

Many backers of this diet suggest that people monitor the pH value of their urine using pH testing strips, to make sure that it is alkaline (pH over 7) and not acidic (under 7). However, it's important to note that the pH value differs greatly within the body. Some parts are alkaline, whereas others are acidic. There is no set level. Unlike many other eccentric diets, the alkaline diet is actually pretty healthy and balanced. It encourages a high consumption of vegetables, fruits, and healthy plant based foods, whilst minimizing processed junk foods.

Acids are actually some of the most important building blocks of the body, including; DNA (deoxyribonucleic acid), fatty acids, and amino acids.

The alkaline diet is healthy because it is based on real and not processed foods that are abundant in the western world. It has absolutely nothing to do with being alkaline or acidic. It's just how your body reacts to the food.

Alkaline Diet Guidelines

Acid-promoting and toxic foods consist of meats, refined carbs, poultry, and dairy. These foods create the kind of acidic environment in your body that puts stress on the liver and kidney, and can put you in the risk category for diabetes. Foods that produce alkaline segments in the body though, help to neutralize those effects. Knowing which foods promote acidity and which promote alkalinity, is the first step to balancing out your diet.

What to eat

Like any other specialized diet, this too has its restrictions and we will be walking you through them step by step whenever you get confused or forget, this will be a good guide for you to follow later on as well.

Meat, seafood, eggs, vegetables, some fruit (as some of these also contain lots of good sugar needed for your body to electrolyze and hydrate when combined with salt and water), oils, nuts, and seeds. When shopping for your groceries- keep in mind this simple rule - if you can't pronounce it, **DON'T EAT IT**, as lots of nasties are hidden behind good looking packaging and known brands. Stick to simple, single ingredient foods, whole foods, or ones that show no ingredients as these will be the most natural and unprocessed of foods.

Including more of these 21 foods into your diet could drastically help to boost organ health and reduce body weight. The foods listed are from most neutral to most alkaline-promoting.

Alkaline-promoting foods:

- Green beans
- Asparagus
- Red wine
- White wine
- Broccoli
- Cauliflower
- Marmalade
- Cherries
- Apples
- Watermelon
- Zucchini
- Hazelnuts
- Tomatoes
- Spinach
- Potatoes
- Bananas
- Apricots
- Radishes
- Carrots
- Celery
- Raisins (most alkaline-promoting)

Recent studies suggest that eating too many acidity promoting foods could potentially harm your liver and kidney, and might even raise your risk of diabetes.

Below you'll find common acid-promoting foods, which are listed from neutral to most acid-forming. If you see some of your favorite foods on this list, you don't need to get rid of them entirely. Instead, neutralize the effects of the acidity with the previous list of alkalizing foods.

Acid-promoting foods:

(Listed from neutral to most acid-forming)

- Lentils, boiled
- Plain bagel
- Whole-wheat cooked spaghetti
- Peanuts, dry-roasted
- White bread
- Walnuts
- Hot dog
- Wild cooked trout
- Pepperoni
- Chicken
- Lean beef
- Whole milk
- Whole egg, hard boiled
- Oats
- White canned tuna fish
- Brown rice
- Cooked salmon
- Cooked turkey bacon
- Mozzarella
- Canned sardines
- Parmesan cheese (most acid-producing)

- American/cheddar cheese
- Low-fat yogurt

What to avoid or eat less often

A few off-limits foods to keep in mind when partaking in this diet include; tortillas, pancakes, bread, muffins, biscuits, cupcakes, waffles, cookies, pizza crust, cereal, French fries, and potato chips this one recipe where eggs, coconut milk, and date paste are combined to create a thick, creamy concoction that can once again transform your undrinkable black coffee into sweet, dreamy caffeine. Use your best judgment with foods that aren't on this list, but that you suspect are not helping you change your habits or break those cravings.

Sugar: Of any kind be it real or artificial (maple syrup, honey, coconut sugar, splenda, equal, nutrasweet, stevia, etc.) Make sure to read your labels and again if you're unsure of what an ingredient in something is, pass it as it is probably in the can't list.

Grains: Such as wheat, oats, corn, and sorghum. This also includes the morning bran or germ shakes. Again - READ YOUR LABELS, to see what each one contains.

Legumes or beans (with a few exceptions): This also includes peanuts, peanut butter, and soy, be it soy sauce, edamame.

Dairy: No cow, goat, or sheep products including creams, milks, cheeses, ice creams, or yogurt of any kind.

The reasons behind the food breakdowns why vs. why not.

In this diet you can't eat grains, dairy, or sugar. Let's look a little closer as to WHY NOT.

Sugar

Sugar contains a whole bunch of calories that we call empty – they contain NO essential nutrients. There are no proteins, essential fats or minerals in it. It contributes to diabetes and obesity.

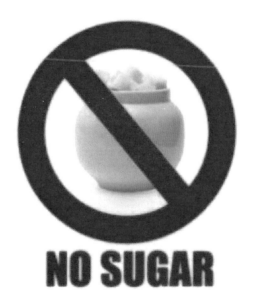

NO SUGAR

It contains two forms of simple sugars: glucose and fructose.

Glucose is found in every living cell therefore if we don't get it somewhere our bodies will naturally produce it (therefore we do not need to add more to our bodies.

Fructose can ONLY be metabolized by the liver and only in very specific amounts (therefore if we intake too much it does not get processed properly). Meaning if we overload our system with fructose it overloads the liver causing it to turn it into fat. This can lead to disease such as fatty liver. It can also cause an insulin resistance. Insulin is a very important hormone within our bodies which allows glucose (blood sugar) to enter cells from the bloodstream and tells the cells to burn glucose instead of fat. Too much glucose in the blood can cause diabetes and blindness. The metabolic dysfunction caused by the "western diet" is that insulin stops working as it should and the cells become resistant to it.

Dairy

Dairy - well, there are now a lot of research that states dairy isn't all it's cracked up to be. We have grown up stating that milk and dairy will help with brittle bones however it is scientifically proven that countries that have the least intake of dairy products such as Africa and Asia have the lowest rates of osteoporosis.

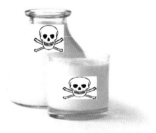

Studies on calcium itself now even state that vitamin D plays a bigger role in helping with bone health than calcium. Especially since people in sun starved countries or people that layer themselves in sun cream (which prevents UV B – vitamin D and not UV A – damaging rays) think that it will substitute for lack of sun but it won't because you need vitamin D to absorb the nutrients you consume every day. It is even stated that the FTC recently asked the USDA to look at their scientific claims because milk does not increase sports performance and there's no evidence that dairy PREVENTS osteoporosis.

Plus, it's loaded with saturated fats which lead to heart disease.

Grains

Grains - well there, this one too is a good one. We are all told to eat a whole grain diet when in all actuality at this point in this ever evolving world of sustenance, it may not be the best thing for you. The way grains are milled in modern time allows shelf stable foods to be manufactured many months in advance of distribution. It also eliminates the richest source of the proteins, vitamins and lipids found in grains such as bran germ and shorts. The replacements used in factories are without their whole food complex. The finding of what percentage found to be lost in modern industrial processing is usually over 70% and always over 50%. We now also have to fight with hybrid seeds, modern irrigation techniques and the synthetic fertilizers used to grow such crops.

Let's also talk about the pesticides and chemicals used as well. These all create a new species of crop and also can contribute to intake health issues.

Fielding crops in the manner we do with modern advances sometimes creates biological manipulation and issue resistant strains being harvested (pests, drought, and blight). Let's step away from just the crop for a second and look deeper into what sort of soil they are planted in and what sort of irrigation they are maintained with. Easier harvests yes, but at what cost to you the consumer?

All of these issues play a part in health issues and disease, as they are seen as true foreign estrogens in our bodies and we are not created or genetically equipped to properly fully digest them.

7 Day Meal Plan

Day 1:

Breakfast – Buckwheat Porridge

Lunch – Swiss Chard Wrap

Dinner – Quinoa Salad with Grilled Red Peppers and Spiralized Vegetables

Dessert – Apple and Peanut Butter Sarnies

Day 2:

Breakfast – Super Detox Breakfast Smoothie

Lunch – Mediterranean Alkaline Pasta

Dinner – Alkaline Vegetable Stir-Fry with Kohlrabi & Leeks

Dessert – Lemon and Berry Cheesecake

Day 3:

Breakfast – Savory Pancakes

Lunch – Black Bean Quinoa Salad

Dinner – Chickpeas & Zucchini Sauce

Dessert – Creamed Spinach

Day 4:

Breakfast – Avocado Smash on Toast

Lunch – Stuffed Cucumbers

Dinner – Gingery Leafy Greens Stir-Fry

Dessert – Nutty Date Rolls

Day 5:

Beet Quinoa with a Hint of Orange

Lunch – Nuts About Salad

Dinner – Broccoli, Carrots & Peas in Coconut Curry Sauce

Dessert – Chocolate Mousse

Day 6:

Breakfast – Tapioca Crêpes

Lunch – Carrot and Goji Berry Soup

Dinner – Avocado & Quinoa Salad

Dessert – Ambercup Coconut Milk Dessert

Day 7:

Breakfast - Granola Swirl

Lunch – Chilled Green Goddess Soup

Dinner – Roasted Garbanzo Bean Curry Salad

Dessert – Chocolate Oranges

Conclusion

While it is extremely important to eat well, you must keep in mind that, to achieve a clean eating lifestyle, one must keep a positive attitude. No matter how well you eat, it will only keep your body in good shape, if your mind is not healthy. Exercise every day, not only to work off any extra calories, but to keep your body lithe and well, and your mind clear. Keeping yourself in good health and in a happy mood will invite those around you to smile more and join you in your journey.

Cooking has never been more diverse, making it near impossible for any picky eater to dislike the food through and through. There will be more and more ways of cooking everything, and new ingredients will emerge. All this enables you to facilitate a transition into a healthier life filled with a variety of food that comes from the four corners of the world. Meal planning will inadvertently reduce stress in one aspect of your life, as well as planning your grocery shop. Clean eating will reduce the risks of many illnesses and increase the likelihood of a longer, happier life, and all that is left is to give yourself the first push to start. A nutritious, well-balanced, diverse diet, along with lots of exercise, shying away from smoking anything and not drinking excessively are the basics of obtaining and maintaining good health.

The benefits of adopting the alkaline diet are; you'll be more fulfilled and less hungry, I know this because whenever I eat more than usual one day I'm usually just as hungry the next day too, as my stomach has expanded to meet the amount of food I was eating the previous day thus adapting itself for today and making my appetite as big as yesterday's. You'll reduce your risk of illnesses and diseases by keeping your body's pH levels neutral. If you train yourself to eat a certain way, your body will get used to it, and eating the right amounts will leave you feeling less hungry, your health will reflect in your energy levels by it being increased, your skin will start to glow and your blood cells will renew itself with healthy nutrients rather than toxins infusing into the blood and tissues from bad processed food. Furthermore, bones renew themselves every 10 years and what you eat vastly affects the health of those new bones that you are contributing to by what you eat because your bone tissue absorbs it.

Suppress your wants and give into your needs, you'll be doing yourself a favor and your future self will thank you. When it comes to eating healthier, quality trumps quantity.

Eat a balanced diet

Eating healthily will reduce the risk of some types of cancers and diseases, not only that but if you get sick often, it most likely isn't due to the environment you are exposed to but your current diet because many fresh foods have bacteria fighting properties in them. For example; eating citrusy fruits like; kiwis, oranges, lemons, and limes (in your water/fresh juices) give acidity to your stomach, liver and bladder which helps fight ulcers and infections if and when they occur.

Proteins are a vital part of our diet to build and maintain muscle and body weight. So, instead of going for the most obvious proteins; red meats, steaks, etc. change it to plant based proteins or sustainable and environmentally friendly fish as this doesn't only benefit the environment but also your health. Fish is also known as brain food because of its omega 3 & 6 content, however bare in mind the type of fish you choose at the store because most fish have a higher content of omega 6 and less of the omega 3, which most people are deficient in. Fish with a high content of omega 3 include; kipper fillets and sardines. In this day and age eating organic is all the craze and this is why; strict laws have been put in place about the labelling of organic products which keeps profit crazed companies from adding chemicals to your food. Don't be fooled by a product that states that it has all natural ingredients because when a consumer reads 'natural' on a product label they expect plant-based ingredients only, little do they know the food could be grown with pesticides as it is cheaper than natural fertilizer. Labelling regulations on the word 'natural' is less strict because there is no more meaning to natural.

Fun fact: What we eat has an impact on our brains. Did you know that bananas contain 10 milligrams of dopamine, an awesome mood booster for the brain? Dark chocolate, packed with polyphenol, is also known to boost serotonin, a neurotransmitter that many antidepressants greatly target.

Do not snack after dinner

If you get hungry; grab a piece of fruit. Smart, simple and healthy choices like replacing soda with homemade juice (made from fresh ingredients, which can be store in the fridge), baking homemade vegetables like; pumpkin, squash or carrot strips, instead of eating packaged crisps that are heavy in saturated fat, are a great low fat choice. When eating out, ordering a side of salad instead of fries will suppress the urge to snack as it does not fluctuate, causing blood cholesterol levels to fluctuate making your body crave more.

Avoid highly processed and sugary foods

They will bring you nothing but a physiological high and a physical low. As Your body has to work really hard to balance your body levels again. So, when blood sugar is high it causes you to want to continue eating to stay on the high, so it doesn't fluctuate cause body levels to fluctuate from a high to a low dramatically.

Pre-packaged foods like ready meals, that you can just bung in the microwave as is, is the worst kind of processed food there is because they add so many more chemicals that are toxins to your body in order to make it look more appealing and to sustain flavor and durability while in the store. Unhealthy food also takes a toll on your metabolism to get rid of excess in the body from food that it doesn't need by storing it as fat. So, if you eat too many processed foods the metabolism will start to deteriorate as it cannot keep up with the workload and as your metabolism fails on you so will the balance in body levels, the metabolism tries to sustain.

Success Stories

"True change comes when you have a choice, a choice of walking through two doors. Which door is less painful to walk through...the first door of continuing those familiar current habits and suffering the painful health consequences alongside

I knew the value of going raw; I had a water alkalizer, even a case of pH paper to check myself. I'd check myself a lot, try to do a lot of things but could never get myself alkaline. That was the day I started reading up on the alkaline diet and pH values. I learned where my weaknesses are that stopped me from alkalizing (one acidic muffin a day is a no-no), what huge gaps I had. For 53 years I prided myself for never using salt, for being a long-term athlete and no salt. My coach showed how wrong I was and why. I added alkaline sea salts, salt to my program, upped my oils to a quart a week. I read and re-read each chapter till I really understood what to do.

I made the commitment to the most alkalizing energizing food source, the healthiest food possible for my body, I wanted to be a pH Miracle Man!"

Rick Laurenzi

"I've been eating a keto diet for 3 months. I'm a 55 yr old 1st grade teacher. After the first month, I realized my legs were no longer swollen all the time. I then realized I was no longer taking aspirin/ibuprofen at least once, and usually twice, per day. My energy levels are going up. My weight is dropping slowly, but surely. I feel better than I have in years. This is no longer a 'diet'. It's a new way of life. I won't go back. I've cheated twice during the past 3 months. Both times, I ate a cookie and quickly felt awful. That awful feeling lasted 3 days! I was hoping the first cheat/feeling awful incident was a coincidence. The second cheat showed me it wasn't. I know I will be diabetic or worse if I don't remain on this new way of eating. I am at peace with this. I will be fine and look forward to my feeling good/healthy future."

Sarah Barker Stewart

"14 days just cutting to 20 net carbs, and eliminating added sugar! Without even tracking religiously I am down around 16 pounds, 5 inches off my waist, hips and bust each!!!!) my migraines have stopped and I have so much more energy and better sleep! My libido along with my confidence have soared, and I am incredibly sorry that I didn't start this months ago! If you're reading this, START NOW! Or you'll be wishing you did"

Erin Ward

Hello Dear Reader:

Thanks for buying my book. I hope this note finds you in good health and that the information in this book is helping you to feel fabulous every day.

My apologies for interrupting your reading, but I want to ask you a favor. If this book has inspired you to take some steps toward improving your health, or just to cook up some new recipes, please go to Amazon and leave me a review.

And if you have comments, suggestions, or questions, please email me directly at eric.p.garvin@gmail.com and I will try to incorporate your feedback before the next reprint is issued.

Have a great day and be healthy!

Sincerely,
Eric Garvin

Breakfast Recipes

Avocado Smash on Toast

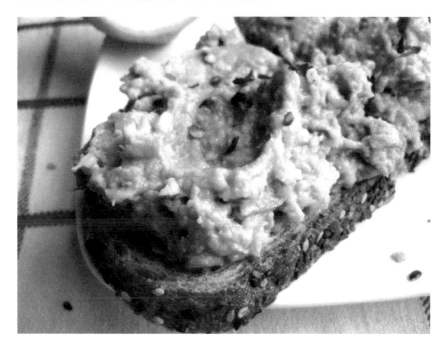

Avocados are a known superfood, and with good reason! These green gems are packed with vitamin E, an essential nutrient for clear, healthy, and glowing skin. They're perfect for breakfast as they are both creamy and filling, setting you up perfectly for the day ahead. Avocados can be tricky in terms of judging how ripe they are and when to slice into them. You can gage whether your avocados are ready for use by gently squeezing one with your hand. If the avocado squashes slightly, it is ready to eat. Do not use hard avocados for this recipe as you will end up with a bitter tasting topping!

This recipe works brilliantly on any kind of toast, although if you couple this idea with homemade sourdough bread, you'll find a new level of appreciation.

Ingredients

- ½ avocado
- Coconut or vegetable spread
- Sundried tomato or olives (optional)
- Marmite or vegemite (optional)
- Seasoning (sea salt, ground black pepper)

Method

Toast your bread in the grill or toaster.

Slice the avocado in half using a bread knife and scoop out ¼ of the flesh into a bowl.

Mash the avocado using a fork and season.

Spread a layer of coconut spread, marmite or vegemite onto your toast (optional).

Spoon the avocado smash onto the toast and top with sundried tomatoes and olives (optional).

Tofu Scramble

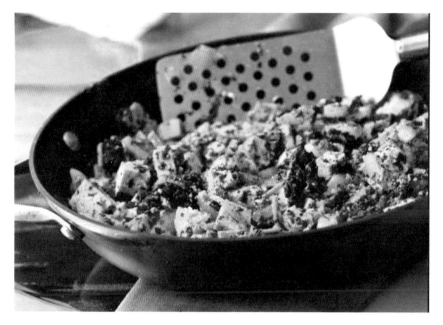

A quick and easy alternative to scrambled eggs, tofu scramble is a great way to get a portion of protein into your body for breakfast. This recipe can be jazzed up by adding your favorite combination of herbs, olives, sundried tomatoes, nuts and spices. You can serve tofu scramble individually or on toast.

Ingredients

- 1-2 cups firm tofu
- extra virgin olive oil
- 1 clove of garlic
- Sundried tomato or olives (optional)
- Mushrooms and baby spinach (optional)
- Seasoning (sea salt, ground black pepper, turmeric, basil)

- Organic soy milk

Method

Lightly heat up your frying pan with a drizzle of vegetable oil and fry your garlic with any additional spices (turmeric provides a bright yellow coloring for aesthetic appeal).

Remove tofu from packaging, rinse under cold water and place between a few sheets of kitchen roll.

Gently squeeze the tofu to remove additional water.

Throw tofu into the frying pan and break into pieces with a spatula.

Add any additional veggies such as mushrooms or baby spinach leaves.

Season with your desired herbs and toppings.

Fry on a medium heat for around 5 – 8 minutes, allowing the tofu to brown slightly on the edges.

Serve alone or on toast.

Super Detox Breakfast Smoothie

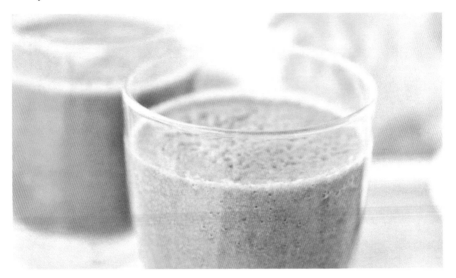

This healthy breakfast detox smoothie helps your body keep sugar cravings at minimum. It's packed with antioxidants, vitamins, and alkalizing minerals. It's very tasty too!

Ingredients

- 1 whole lemon, juiced
- ½ cup chopped cucumber
- 1 cup chopped romaine leaves
- 1 cup chopped kale or spinach
- ½ tbsp. chia seeds
- 1 small pear (or ½ large), cored and chopped
- 1 avocado, chopped
- ½ cup chopped celery
- 1 cup coconut water
- 1 tbsp. fresh parsley
- 1 tbsp. fresh mint

- ¼-inch slice ginger root, peeled

Method

Blend together all ingredients in a blender until very smooth. Enjoy!

Strawberry and Avocado Smoothie

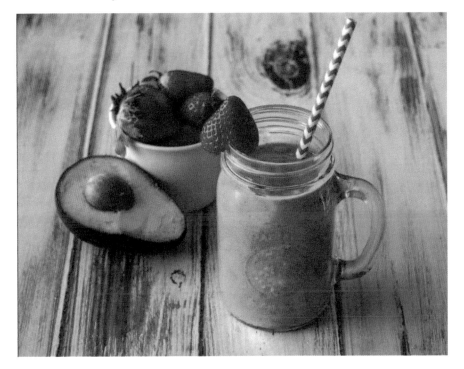

This is an awesome alkalizer smoothe that will delight everyone. Create vibrant health and restore energy with this super healthy pH-balancing alkaline smoothie.

Ingredients

- ½ avocado, chopped
- 200ml almond milk
- 4 tbsp. nonfat Greek yogurt
- 150g strawberries, halved
- 1 tbsp. freshly squeezed lemon juice

Method

Put all the ingredients in a blender and whizz until smooth. If the consistency is too thick, add a little water.

Beet Quinoa with a Hint of Orange

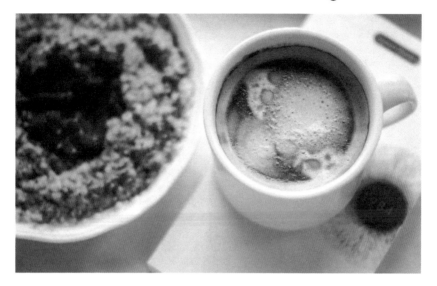

The creativity in this recipe marries the beautiful red color of beets with the sweetness of orange. This dish will be a treat for the eyes and taste buds, and your family will love it!

Ingredients

- ½ red onion thinly sliced
- 1 tablespoon apple cider vinegar
- 2-3 beets
- 1 cup quinoa
- 1 stalk celery, thinly sliced
- 1 teaspoon grated ginger
- Extra virgin olive oil
- Juice of 1 lemon
- 1 small orange, thinly sliced
- ½ tsp. sea salt
- ½ tsp. freshly ground black pepper

Method

Combine sliced onion and apple cider vinegar in a bowl; let soak for at least 10 minutes.

In the meantime, bring a pot of water to a gentle boil over medium heat. Rinse the beets and add to the boiling water; boil for about 10 minutes or until tender cooked, but not mushy.

Transfer the beets to a plate and reserve the cooking liquid;peel the cooked beets and chop thinly.

Follow package instructions to cook quinoa using the reserved beet liquid. Season with salt while cooking. When cooked, remove the quinoa from heat and set aside to cool.

In a large serving bowl, mix beets, quinoa, ginger and celery. Remove onion from the vinegar and stir into the bowl with the quinoa mixture.

Drizzle with extra virgin olive oil and lemon juice. Add orange slices and toss to mix well.

Season with salt and pepper to serve.

Buckwheat Porridge

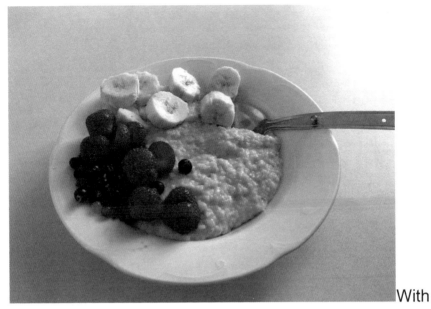

With a wonderful nutty flavor, buckwheat is a gluten-free, low GI seed that is high in fiber, amino acids and essential minerals. The fiber is buckwheat is soluble thus helps promote bowel health and reduce blood cholesterol levels. Buckwheat is also a good source of antioxidant, anti-inflammatory polyphenols, such as rutin, which aids in reducing blood pressure. Chia seeds in this recipe boost the omega 3. A touch of cinnamon will boost the flavor of porridge and also help reduce blood sugar.

Ingredients

- ½ cup roasted buckwheat
- pinch cinnamon
- 1 cup almond milk
- 2 tablespoons chia seed
- 1 teaspoon vanilla

- small handful large raisins
- 1 red apple, grated
- Dried goji and fresh blueberries to serve

Method

In a large bowl, mix buckwheat, cinnamon, milk, chia, vanilla,and raisins; stir and refrigerate for at least 8 hours or overnight. Stir in grated apple and cook over medium-low heat for about 5 minutes or until creamy and thick. Add more milk if necessary.

Serve porridge in bowls topped with goji and blueberries.

Savory Pancakes

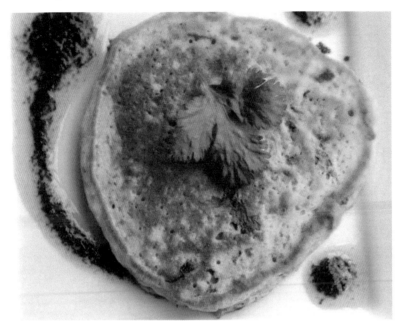

These savory chickpea pancakes are a high protein, sugar-free alternative to the conventional breakfast treat. They can be topped with avocado, salad, fried peppers, wilted spinach and any other veggies. These pancakes will keep you going through till the afternoon and are the perfect flavorful kick starter for your day.

Ingredients

- Spring onions (chopped finely)
- ¼ cup Red Bell Peppers (chopped finely)
- 1 clove garlic
- ½ cup Besan (chickpea) flour
- ¼ teaspoon sea salt (finely ground)
- Water
- Toppings: Guacamole, salsa, hummus etc.

Method

Lightly heat frying pan and prepare veggies.

Whisk up the flour, seasoning and baking powder in a small bowl.

Add in ½ cup of water and mix until smooth, creating air bubbles.

Stir the chopped vegetables through.

Drizzle oil onto pan and pour batter to make one pancake.

Cook on each side for around 5 minutes and flip when browned.

Serve hot with toppings.

Granola Swirl

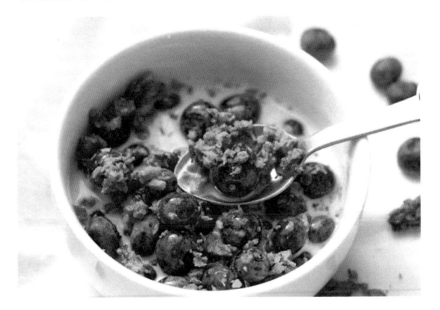

This super quick and easy recipe can be made up in one glass, within 5 minutes! It is also packed with calcium, protein and antioxidants. This combination can be adapted with your favorite fruits and nuts, providing a different range of flavors and nutrients every time. If you have spare time on your hands, you can also stew apple, sugar and water to provide a deeper layer of taste and satisfaction. Served in a glass to display the layers, this stunning breakfast is one you won't forget!

Ingredients

- ½ handful blueberries
- ½ cup granola
- Dairy-free yoghurt
- Agave nectar
- 2 pitted dates

Method

Layer a glass with a spoonful of dairy free yoghurt.

Add a spoonful of granola.

Add a layer of chopped dates and blueberries.

Repeat the layering process and finish with the yoghurt.

Swirl on the agave nectar for the finishing touch of sweetness.

Tapioca Crêpes

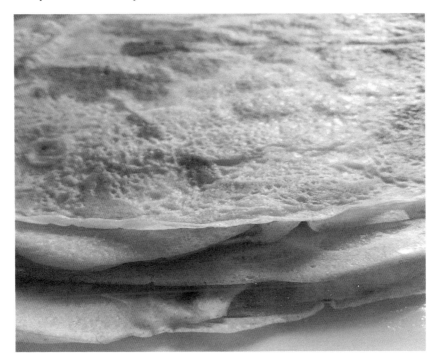

Yields: 2 Servings

Total Time: 35 Minutes

Prep Time: 10 Minutes

Cook Time: 25 Minutes

Ingredients

- 1 large free range egg
- 1 cup full fat coconut milk
- 1 cup tapioca flour
- 1/4 tsp. sea salt
- Toppings of choice- for crepes, (I prefer almond butter and berries, but you can also mix it up with cinnamon, applesauce, sautéed veggies, etc.)

Method

In a medium bowl, mix together all the ingredients.

Set a skillet over medium heat and add 1/3 cup of the mixture when hot, tilting the skillet to spread out the batter.

Cook both sides for about 4 minutes or until lightly browned.

Serve warm topped with desired ingredients.

Lunch Recipes

Mediterranean Alkaline Pasta

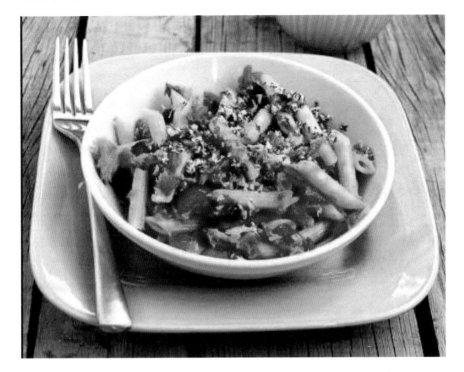

This vibrant lunchtime dish is the perfect partner for a packed lunch! It takes just under 20 minutes to prepare and can be made up in batches that could be stored in a fridge or even frozen for times when you don't have the chance to cook up something fresh.

Ingredients

- Spelt pasta
- 1 bell pepper (or ½ of two color variations)
- ½ cup olives (pitted)
- 1 clove of garlic
- ¼ cup of extra virgin olive oil
- ½ cup of roasted almonds (roughly chopped)

- Seasoning (basil, salt pepper)
- 1 red onion (finely chopped)
- Handful of fresh thyme
- 1 tbsp. yeast flakes

Method

Boil and cook the spelt pasta as instructed on packaging.

Heat up a frying pan with oil.

Fry the garlic and onion for 5 minutes.

Chop and prepare the veggies.

Cook veggies in the pan with the garlic and onion, until slightly charred.

Once pasta is cooked, drain using a sieve and rinse to remove any starch.

Season veggies and serve up the pasta, top with veggies and a drizzle of olive oil.

Chop up the thyme leaves and sprinkle on top.

Add some yeast flakes to your dish for additional flavor (optional).

Nuts About Salad

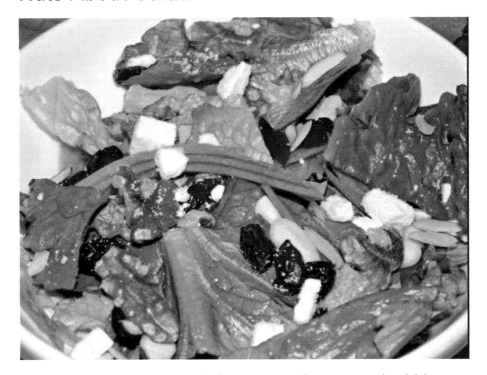

Who says that vegan salads are pure leaves and rabbit food? You can enhance the nutritional value of any green salad by throwing in some nuts and seeds. This recipe tosses the conventional salad rules out of the window – Prepare your taste buds!

Ingredients

- Rocket Lettuce
- Iceberg Lettuce
- Baby Spinach Leaves
- Sweet bell pepper
- Cos Lettuce
- 1 orange (peeled and sliced into small chunks)

- Trail mix
- Olive oil
- Basil leaves (fresh)
- Lemon Juice (1/2 lemon)
- Grated carrot
- ¼ cup sultanas
- Seasoning (ground black pepper)
- Hummus (optional)

Method

Prepare the dressing by combining olive oil, fresh basil leaves and lemon juice.

Wash all of the salad ingredients thoroughly and leave to drain.

Once the leaves have drained, mix them together in a large bowl, creating the bed of the salad.

Season with ground black pepper.

Add in thin slices of the sweet bell pepper and grated carrot.

Mix in the orange slices (apple slices may also be used) and sultanas.

Pour the dressing and toss the salad.

Sprinkle the trail mix over the salad before serving.

Serve with hummus (optional).

Stuffed cucumber

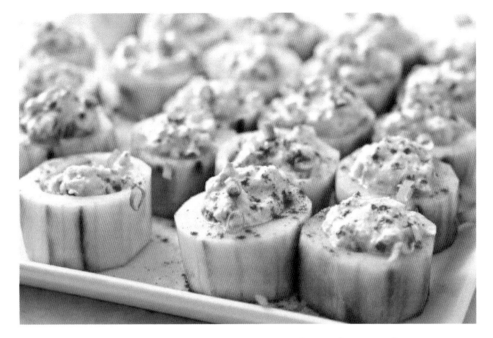

This neat recipe involves the preparation of a mock tuna salad, served and presented in slices of cucumber. As the almonds require soaking for optimum softness (6-8 hours), be sure to plan this meal the night before.

Ingredients

- 1 clove garlic (mashed)
- 1 cup almonds (raw and soaked)
- 2 stalks celery (finely chopped)
- 2 spring onions (finely chopped)
- 3 tablespoons vegan mayonnaise
- 1 teaspoon mustard (Dijon)
- Seasoning (black pepper, sea salt, lemon juice)
- 1 large cucumber (chopped into 1cm thick rounds)

Method

Grind up the almonds in a food processor to create the 'tuna' flakes and add to mixing bowl.

Throw in all of the filling ingredients and mix together.

Use a teaspoon to scoop out the innards of the cucumber, creating a small hole in the center of each round.

Season the cucumber and scoop the filling into the hole.

Serve as a platter or try out the mixture in a wrap, pitta or with salad leaves for future variation.

Black Bean Quinoa Salad

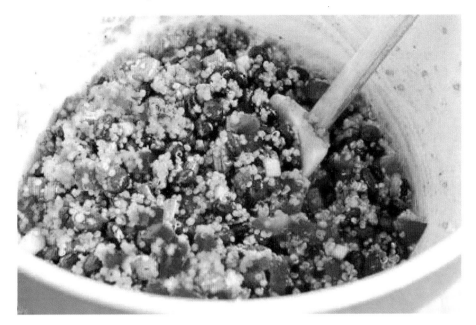

This high protein salad is made up of beans and grains rather than pure salad leaves. This dish is gluten-free and can also be made with other grains or couscous, depending on your preference. You may even decide to mix things up on the next level and combine different grains for added taste and texture.

Ingredients

- ½ cup pine nuts
- 1 ½ cups quinoa (or other preferred grains)
- 2 Roma tomatoes (finely diced and peeled)
- 1 cucumber (English, finely diced)
- ½ red onion (finely chopped)
- ¼ cup extra virgin olive oil
- 1 can black beans

- ½ cup fresh parsley (finely chopped)
- 2 teaspoons lemon zest (grated finely)
- 3 tablespoons lemon juice

Method

Pre-heat oven to 400 degrees Fahrenheit.

Prepare quinoa or grains as instructed.

Lay out a baking sheet onto the baking tray.

Sprinkle pine nuts onto tray and brown them in the oven for a couple of minutes.

Rinse out the canned black beans and add to mixing bowl.

When browned, throw the nuts into the mixing bowl and add in all of the other ingredients.

Make up the dressing and stir through.

This dish can be served as a hot or cold salad.

Chilled Green Goddess Soup

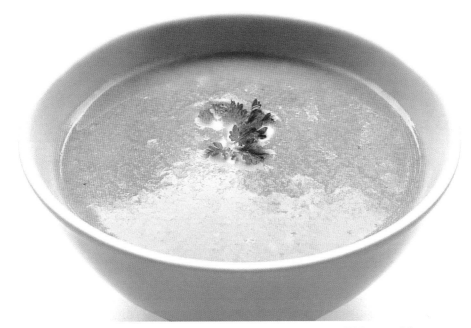

This is a vibrant green soup that everyone will love. You may want to add even more flavor to this soup by drizzling runny tahini and sprinkling some toasted nuts and seeds when serving.

Ingredients

- 6 cups (1350 grams) cucumber
- 2 stalks celery chopped
- 1-2 cups water (depending how thin you want it)
- 2 tablespoons fresh lime juice
- 1 cup (225 grams) watercress leaves
- 1 cup (225 grams) rocket leaves
- ½ cup (120 grams)mashed avocado (roughly 1 avocado)

- 1 teaspoon wheatgrass power or a mixed green powder, optional
- Sea salt to taste

Method

Blend all ingredients except the avocado in a blender until a broth forms. Strain the liquid through a cheesecloth or fine sieve. Then return to blender and add the avocado and blend until smooth.

Garnish with a few watercress leaves and cracked black pepper.

Swiss Chard Wrap

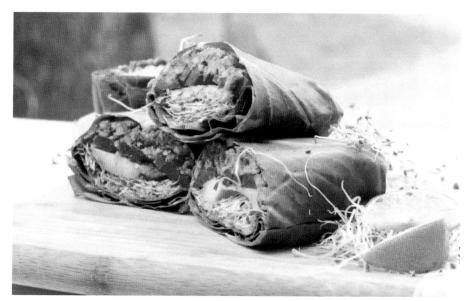

Try using the greens for the wraps and the white bottoms thinly sliced added to the filling, for added nutrition with your wrap. One of the dark, leafy greens that nutritionists frequently recommend, Swiss chard is similar to spinach, kale and collard greens. Tall and leafy with a crunchy stalk, chard is slightly salty and a tad bitter, and works well with fish and vegetable dishes. But what makes chard so compelling is its nutritional profile.

Chard is an excellent source of vitamins A, K, C, E, magnesium, manganese, potassium and iron.

A good choice to lower cancer risk. Its combination of minerals, phytonutrients and fiber may help to prevent digestive tract cancers, including colon cancer.

If you are unfamiliar with chard, try substituting it in recipes that call for fresh spinach or other greens.

Experiment with seasonings, and you will likely find chard to be a welcome addition to your healthy diet. When choosing Swiss chard, look for stalks and leaves that are paler in color, as white chard tends to be the tenderest. And if you're looking for an easy vegetable to grow, chard needs little care and thrives in almost any climate.

Ingredients

- 4 large swiss chard leaves
- 1 red bell pepper
- 1 avocado
- ¼ -1/3 cups (2-3 ounces) alfalfa sprouts
- 1 carrot
- 1 cucumber
- ½ lime
- 1/4 cup raw pecans
- 1 tablespoon tamari (gluten-free soy sauce)
- 1 teaspoon cumin
- ½ teaspoon minced garlic
- ½ teaspoon grated ginger
- 1 teaspoon olive oil
- Handful of alfalfa sprouts

Method

To prepare Swiss chard, wash leaves, cut off stiff white stem at the bottom and slice thinly to be added to each wrap. Or Juiced! Dry leaves with paper towels; with a knife, thinly slice down the central root.

Thinly slice all the veggies.

In a food processor, combine pecans, tamari, cumin, garlic, ginger and olive oil. Pulse until combined.

Place a collard leaf in front of you and layer nut mix, red pepper slices, avocado slices, cucumber, carrot, alfalfa sprouts, and a dash of lime juice. Then wrap up the sides. You can also use a toothpick to keep the wrap together if it decides to unwrap.

Carrot and Goji Berry Soup

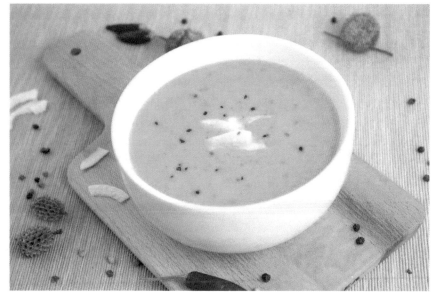

Goji berries are very nutritious and versatile. And this recipe is a must try –it's simply perfection!

Ingredients

- 1 ¼ cups (10 ounces) of fresh carrot juice
- 1 inch ginger, juiced with carrots
- ½ inch turmeric, juiced with carrots
- 1 cup (½ pounds) carrots
- 1 cup (½ pounds) pumpkin
- 2 tablespoon Goji berries
- 2 tablespoons coconut oil
- 1 cup (225 grams)onion, chopped
- 1 red jalapeno pepper-seeds removed
- 2 cups (16 ounces)water
- ½ cup (4 ounces) light coconut milk
- 1 clove garlic

- Sea salt and cracked black pepper to taste

Method

Juice 1 ¼ cups worth of carrots with the turmeric and ginger. Once done, soak the goji berries in the juice for roughly 20 minutes.

Heat coconut oil in a pot and add the onions; sauté for about 4 minutes or until soft, and then add the jalapeno pepper and garlic cook for 1 minute more. Stir in the chopped carrots and water and bring to a boil. Once boiling, reduce heat to a simmer and cook, covered, for about 20 minutes. Cool slightly and transfer the mixture to the blender and add the coconut milk; blend to a thick puree. Strain the goji berries from the carrot juice and set aside.

Add this juice to the puree and continue pureeing until smooth. Season with salt and pepper to taste.

To serve, garnish each serving with of the goji berries.

Dinner Recipes

PB Tofu Slices with a Sauce

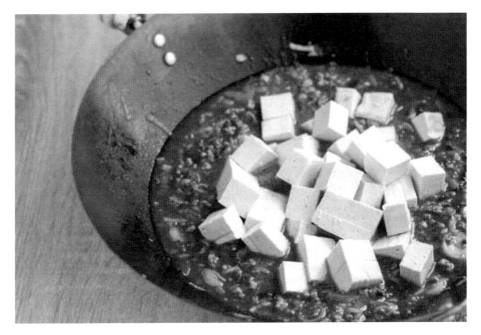

Peanut butter and tofu combined, yes that's right, heaven can exist within the kitchen! Load up on your protein with this rich, spicy and satisfying Asian cuisine inspired meal.

Ingredients

- 3-4 cups firm tofu
- 3 garlic cloves (finely chopped)
- 1 knob ginger (peeled and finely grated)
- 1 tablespoon canola oil (or sesame, avocado, olive sunflower, or coconut oil)1 spring onion (sliced finely for garnishing)
- 3 tablespoons soy sauce (reduced salt)
- 2 tablespoons smooth butter (reduced salt and sugar)

- 3 tablespoons apple cider vinegar tablespoon molasses 2 tablespoons water

Method

Drain out the tofu and squeeze between sheets of kitchen towel to remove excess water.

Make the sauce by whisking the vinegar, soy sauce, peanut butter, water, and agave nectar.

Prepare the spring onion, garlic and ginger.

Heat up the wok and add oil.

Cook the ginger and garlic until fragrant then remove and set aside.

Add the tofu pieces and cook on a medium heat, flipping them over and allowing them to brown on either side (this should take 5-8 minutes).

Once the tofu slices have browned, pour in the sauce and cook until thickening occurs.

Add the garlic and ginger along with the spring onions and garnish.

Season and adjust the sauce flavor if necessary.

Squash Risotto

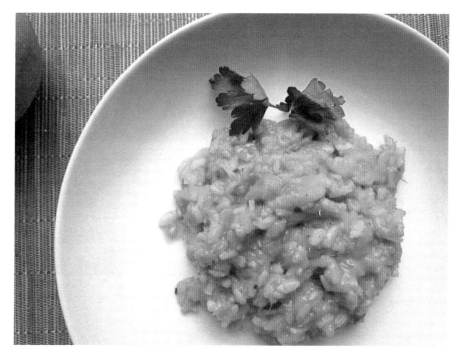

Creamy, vibrant and wholesome – This recipe takes a classic dinner dish (risotto) and combines it with fresh basil, summer squash and peas. It's the perfect meal for those uplifting summer evenings.

Ingredients

- 1 onion (finely chopped)
- 2 tablespoons olive oil
- 2 cloves garlic
- 4 cups vegetable stock
- 1 cup Arborio rice
- ¼ cup white wine
- ½ cup frozen peas (thawed)
- ¼ cup fresh basil leaves

- Ground black pepper
- 1 tablespoon vegan margarine or a dash of dairy free milk

Method

Prepare the squash by washing and slicing into crescents (1 ½ inches thick), set aside.

Heat up a large saucepan with olive oil and add the garlic and onions.

Sauté for 5 minutes on a medium heat.

Stir the rice into the pan and cook for a further 2 minutes.

Add in the white wine and stir gently until the liquid is absorbed.

Add the stock into the pan one ladle at a time.

Stir frequently and allow the liquid to be absorbed before adding more.

After 15 minutes, add in the peas and squash.

Repeat the process of adding water, stirring and cooking for another 5 minutes until the creamy risotto texture is visible.

Remove the pan from the stove and add the margarine and fresh basil leaves.

Stir gently.

Season with pepper, garnish with basil leaves and add a little lemon juice for an added zing!

Greened Mushrooms

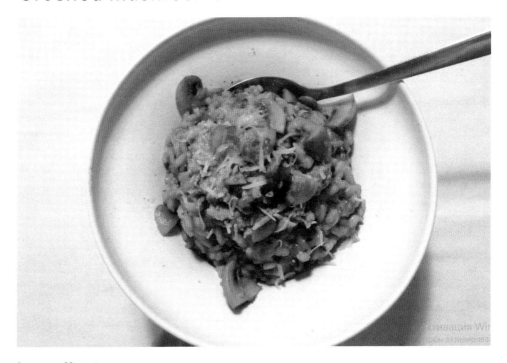

Ingredients

- One 11 oz. package of baby spinach, coarsely chopped
- 1 can green peas
- ½ large onion
- 1 cup mushrooms
- 2-3 tbsp. avocado oil or olive oil
- ½ tsp garlic powder
- Sea salt to taste

Method

In a large sauté pan, on a medium heat, cook the onions in avocado or olive oil.

When they are browned, add in the mushrooms and cook until the mushrooms soften.

Then add the spinach, sea salt and garlic powder, turn down the heat and cover.

Lastly add the green peas and cook for another couple of minutes.

Serve over cooked brown rice

Quinoa Salad with Grilled Red Peppers and Spiralized Vegetables

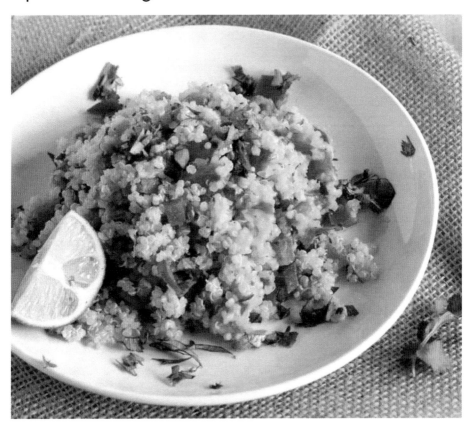

Ingredients

Basil and Green Onion Vinaigrette

- ½ tbsp. olive oil
- ¼ tbsp. lemon juice
- 2 cloves garlic, chopped finely
- ¼ tbsp. chopped green onions
- ¼ tbsp. fresh basil, chopped finely
- Salt and black pepper, to taste

Quinoa Salad

- 1 cup. water
- 1 cup quinoa
- 1 tbsp. olive oil
- 5 mushrooms, sliced
- 1 jar grilled red peppers, cut in strips
- 1 red onion and a carrot cut to the spiralizer
- ¼ cup black olives, sliced

Preparation

For the Vinaigrette:

In a container, put the olive oil, lemon juice, garlic, green onions and basil.

Close the lid and shake. Then season.

Preparation of the salad

Add water to a medium pan and wait until it begins to boil. Add the quinoa and cook for 10 minutes

Drain the quinoa and set aside.

In a frying pan, heat the oil.

Add mushrooms and cook for 3 minutes or until they are soft.

In a salad bowl, mix the quinoa, mushrooms, peppers and onions and carrot in spirals.

Add the vinaigrette and mix delicately to coat the ingredients.

Buckwheat Salad

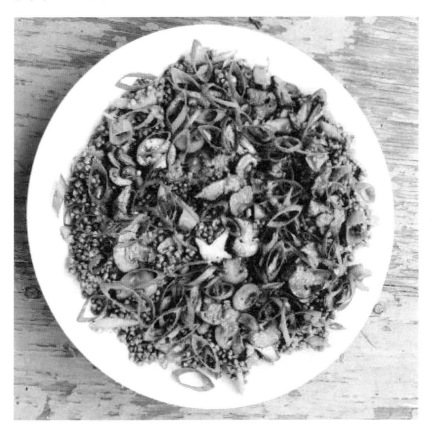

Ingredients

Parsley & Green Onion Vinaigrette

- ½ tbsp. extra virgin olive oil
- ¼ tbsp. of apple cider vinegar
- 2 cloves garlic, chopped finely
- ¼ tbsp. chopped green onions
- ¼ tbsp. fresh basil, chopped finely
- Salt and black pepper to taste

Buckwheat Salad

- 1 cup. water
- 1 cup buckwheat
- 1 tbsp. extra virgin olive oil
- 5 mushrooms, sliced
- 1 red onion and a carrot cut to the spiralizer

Preparation

For the Vinaigrette

In a container, put the olive oil, balsamic vinegar, garlic, green onions and basil.

Close the lid and shake. Then season

Preparation of the salad

Add water to a medium pan and wait until it begins to boil. Add the buckwheat and cook for 10 minutes

Drain the buckwheat and set aside.

In a frying pan, heat the oil.

Add mushrooms and cook for 3 minutes or until they are soft.

In a salad bowl, mix the quinoa, mushrooms and onions and carrot in spirals.

Add the vinaigrette and mix delicately to coat the ingredients.

Spelt Pasta with Eggplant & Zucchini

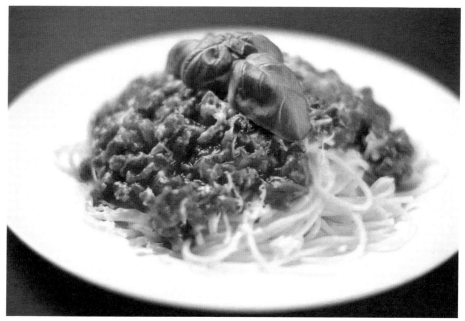

Pasta is a favorite meal to many, yet the "normal" white flour pasta isn't alkaline. Therefore, alkaline spelt pasta, which is usually available in many good grocery stores, will make the best healthy and tasty alternative. The tomato sauce served with this pasta is made with eggplant, zucchini and tomatoes, which are rich sources of alkaline minerals. You can season with favorite herbs for a tasty and filling dinner dish.

Ingredients for 2-3 servings

- 300g spelt pasta
- 3 tbsp. extra virgin olive oil
- 2-3 garlic gloves, crushed
- 1-2 medium white onions, finely diced
- 1 large eggplant, diced

- 1 large zucchini, diced
- 3 medium ripe tomatoes, diced
- 2/3 cup sun dried tomatoes, diced
- 2 tsp. dried basil leaves
- 1 tsp. oregano
- 2/3 cup vegetable broth
- A pinch of Sea salt
- A pinch of pepper
- Fresh basil leaves to serve

Method

Heat oil in a pan over medium heat; sauté garlic, onion and eggplant for about 10 minutes, stirring. Add tomatoes, zucchini and oregano; cook for about 8 minutes more, stirring occasionally.

In the meantime, boil salted water and cook pasta until tender.

Add broth, basil, salt and pepper to the pan and simmer, covered, for a few minutes.

Serve the sauce over the pasta, garnished with fresh basil leaves.

Alkaline Vegetable Stir-Fry with Kohlrabi & Leeks

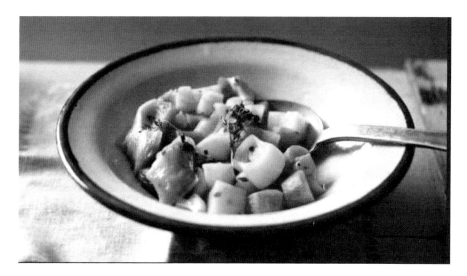

This wonderful vegetable based stir-fry is a real alkaline powerhouse! It's made with interesting herbs, such as dandelion, thyme, and buckhorn plantain, also known as English plantain. It's also filled with richly alkaline green vegetables such as leeks, cabbage, and kohlrabi – also known as German turnip.

Ingredients

- 1 tbsp. butter
- 1 medium white onion, chopped
- 1 big stalk leek, sliced
- 1 small cabbage, chopped
- 3 medium carrots, sliced
- 6 medium potatoes, diced
- 1 kohlrabi with leaves, chopped
- ½ liter vegetable broth

- 1 tsp. thyme
- Dandelion, chopped
- Buckhorn plantain, chopped
- Sea salt
- fresh pepper

Method

Glaze the onion in a frying pan with butter for a few minutes until golden. Stir in all other veggies and broth; cover and simmer for about 15 minutes or until cooked through. Season with thyme, dandelion, buckhorn plantain, salt and pepper. Serve hot.

Buckwheat Pasta with Bell Pepper & Broccoli

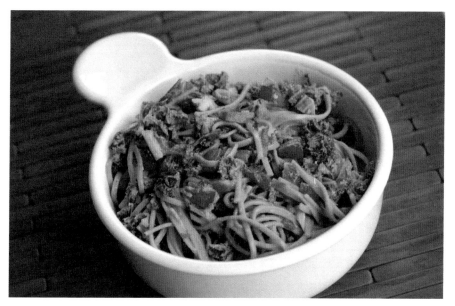

Like spelt, buckwheat pasta is one of the few brands of pasta which are tasty alkaline-friendly pastas. Buckwheat pasta is great when served with fresh alkaline veggies.

Ingredients

- 4 tbsp. olive oil extra virgin
- 500g buckwheat pasta
- 2 garlic cloves, diced
- 1 medium white onion, cut into rings
- 3 carrots, sliced
- 1 head broccoli
- 1 red bell pepper, chopped into strips
- 3 medium tomatoes, diced
- 1 tsp. vegetable broth (yeast free)

- 1 tbsp. fresh lemon juice
- 1 tsp. oregano
- A pinch of Sea salt
- A pinch of pepper

Method

Chop al the veggies read to cook.

Cook buckwheat pasta in boiling salt water. In a separate pot, boil broccoli in boiling salt water.

Meanwhile, heat two tablespoons of oil in a pan and sauté garlic and onion until fragrant and translucent. Remove from pan and set aside.

Heat the remaining oil in the same pan and cook veggies for a few minutes until tender. Add broccoli and onions to the pan and stir in broth, lemon juice, oregano, salt and pepper. Stir to mix well and serve the veggie mix over the buckwheat pasta.

Veggie Stir-Fry with Coconut Milk & Tofu

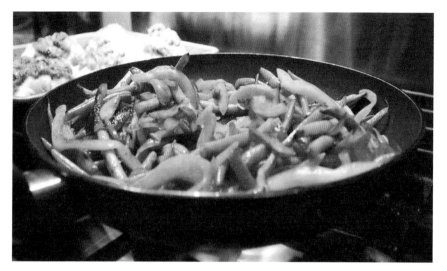

Made from soy beans, tofu is a healthy meat alternative that has an amazing alkaline effect on your body's pH-level.

Ingredients

- ½ pound green beans
- 3 medium zucchinis
- 1 pound firm tofu
- 1 green pepper bell
- 1 red pepper bell
- 3 tomatoes
- 2 tbs. extra virgin olive oil
- 1 ½ cups coconut milk
- ¼ tbs. Ginger
- ½ tbs. curry powder
- A pinch of sea salt and pepper

Method

Dice zucchinis, tofu, bell peppers, tomatoes and beans in bite-size pieces. Heat oil in a pan and fry tofu for about 3 minutes. Add beans, zucchini, and bell peppers; fry for 3 minutes more.

Stir in coconut milk and tomatoes and cook for a few minutes. Season with ginger, curry powder, salt and pepper. Serve with wild rice.

Chickpeas & Zucchini Sauce

This is a very warm, almost raw, filling meal that everyone will love. It's is nutrients-dense and very flavorful. Packed with phyto-nutrients, omega oil and quality protein, this dish is a real alkaline powerhouse. And it's really tasty!

Ingredients

- 1 cup organic vegetable stock (yeast free)
- 120g quinoa
- 400g zucchini, sliced

Sauce Ingredients

- 100g tofu
- 1 tbsp. lemon juice
- ½ tsp. cumin powder
- ½ tsp. chilli powder
- 1 garlic clove
- 400g chick-peas, drained and rinsed
- 2 tbsp. extra virgin olive oil

For serving

- 1 handful fresh parsley, chopped
- 1 large tomato, chopped
- 2 tbsp. toasted sunflower seeds

Method

Cook quinoa in vegetable stock for about 15 minutes or until tender.

Combine all sauce ingredients in a blender and blend until smooth.

Add a small amount of water to a frying pan and steam fry zucchini for about 5 minutes or until tender. Stir in sauce and warm through; stir in olive oil and remove from heat.

Serve the zucchini sauce on two serving platters; top with chopped herbs and tomatoes. Add cooked quinoa and sprinkle with seeds. Enjoy!

Broccoli, Carrots & Peas in Coconut Curry Sauce

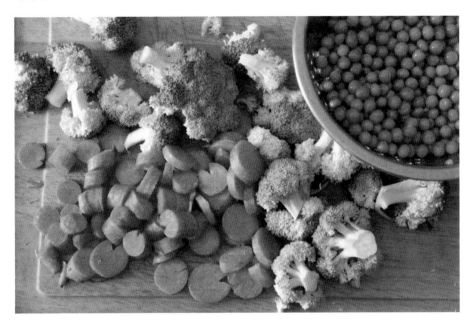

The peas, carrots and broccoli together with curry powder and coconut milk give this meal an abundance of great flavors. Besides the wonderful taste, peas, carrots and broccoli are also nutrient-dense and alkaline, and contain high levels of antioxidants, dietary fiber, vitamin C and minerals.

Ingredients

- 400g carrots, sliced
- 500g broccoli, cut into florets
- 200g fresh peas
- 3 garlic cloves, thinly sliced
- 2 medium onions, thinly sliced
- 200ml vegetable stock (yeast free)

- 200ml coconut milk (unsweetened)
- 2 tbsp. coconut oil
- 1 tbsp. lemon juice
- ½ tsp. grated lemon peel
- 2 tsp. curry powder
- Freshly ground black pepper

Method

Heat two tablespoons of oil in a pan; sauté garlic, onion and curry powder for about 3 minutes.

Add carrots, broccoli, peas, and salt; fry for a few minutes.

Stir in stock, coconut milk, and lemon peel; cover and cook for about 12 minutes.

Serve.

Gingery Leafy Greens Stir-Fry

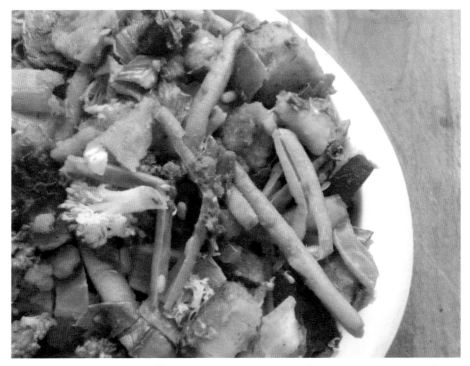

This tasty stir-fry reflects our great love for squashes and pumpkins of all shapes and colors. For the stir-fry, you can use different leafy greens such as spinach, kale, green cabbage, or cavalo nero which are all rich in nutrients and are rich in alkaline minerals. Squashes are also a great source of antioxidants, vitamins, and alkalising minerals.

Ingredients

- 2 tbsp. coconut oil
- 1 onion, finely sliced
- 2-3 garlic cloves, peeled and chopped
- 1 (2-cm) piece of ginger, chopped

- ½ squash, seeded, diced
- 2 handfuls of chopped leafy greens (spinach, kale, or chard)
- 1/4 Savoy cabbage
- 1 red or green chilli, finely chopped
- Fresh juice of ½ a lemon
- A dash of Braggs Liquid Aminos
- A pinch of sea salt
- 1 pinch of freshly ground pepper
- A little water

Method

In a large frying pan set over medium heat, heat coconut oil; sauté onion for about 4 minutes or until fragrant. Stir in garlic, ginger, and chilli; cook for about 5 minutes, stirring. Add squash and salt and cook until squash is tender.

Toss in the leafy green, lemon juice, Braggs Liquid Aminos, salt and pepper; cook for 1 minute.

Avocado & Quinoa Salad

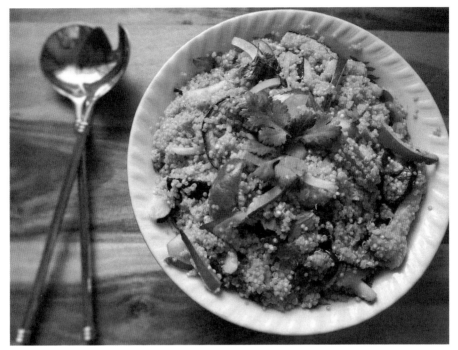

The avocado and quinoa combo in this salad is very addictive. This is a high protein meal with healthy fats from the avocado. It makes a healthy and satisfying meal, perfect for dinner, anytime of your alkaline diet year!

Ingredients

- 1/3 cup quinoa
- 1 avocado, peeled, sliced
- 2 cups baby spinach leaves
- 1/2 tsp. ground cumin seed
- 2 tbsp. lime juice
- 1/4 cup diced red onion
- 1/2 cup diced cucumber
- 1 cup cherry tomatoes, halved

- 2/3 cup water
- Salt

Method

Spread cooked quinoa into a bowl and refrigerate until chilled.

Remove from the refrigerator and stir in onion, cucumber and tomatoes. Season the mixture with salt, cumin seeds, and lime juice. Divide spinach onto serving plates and top each with quinoa salad. To serve, garnish with avocado slices.

Roasted Garbanzo Bean Curry Salad

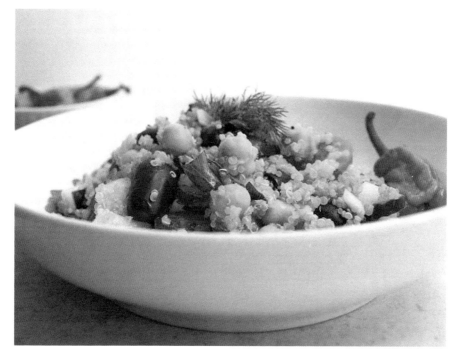

So FRESH and so GOOD! Oven-roasted garbanzo beans add a rich flavor to this salad. If you're not a garbanzo fan, prepare this salad with a different type of beans.

Ingredients

- ½ cup garbanzo beans, rinsed, drained
- 1 tsp. extra virgin olive oil
- ½ cup chopped purple cabbage
- ¼ cup chopped red bell pepper
- ½ cup cooked quinoa
- A pinch of black pepper
- ½ tsp. honey
- 2 tsp. sunflower oil

- ½ tsp. lemon zest
- 2 tsp. freshly squeezed lemon juice
- 1/8 tsp. sea salt
- 1 peeled mandarin orange, chopped
- 1 tbsp. toasted chest nuts

Method

Spread the beans on a baking sheet and bake at 450°F for about 30 minutes or until lightly browned and slightly crunchy. Remove the beans from oven and let cool completely.

Toss together the baked beans, oil, and salt and return to oven for 10 more minutes or until crispy and browned. Remove from oven and let cool.

In a bowl, whisk together sunflower oil, lemon juice, zest, honey, sea salt and black pepper; set aside.

In a bowl, toss together the roasted beans with chopped mandarin orange, red bell pepper, cabbage and cooked quinoa; drizzle with the dressing and sprinkle with toasted chestnuts to serve.

Nutty Date Rolls

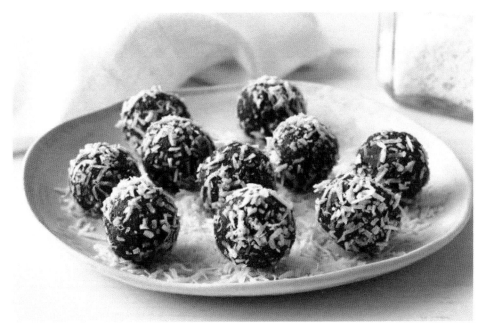

Ingredients

- 1 cup almonds or cashews (raw)
- 1 tablespoon orange juice
- Desiccated coconut flakes
- ¾ cup pitted dates
- Trail mix
- 1 tablespoon almond meal
- 1 tablespoon cinnamon

Method

Place the nuts, dates, trail mix, almond meal and cinnamon into the food processor.

Blend using a grinding blade (add in the orange juice when the blades stick).

Sprinkle the coconut over an area of the worktop.

Shape the mixture into rolls or balls, in the palm of your hand.

Roll the balls in the coconut.

Refrigerate in an airtight container.

Chocolate Mousse

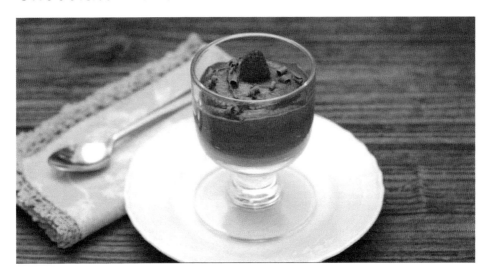

Re-creating the texture of a conventional, diary mousse may sound like a difficult proposition; however the wonders of silken tofu take up the challenge perfectly. These indulgent little desserts can be made and stored in miniature pots and frozen for future sweet tooth cravings.

Ingredients

- 1 cup dark chocolate (dairy free)
- ½ cup maple syrup
- 2 cups silken tofu
- Zest of 1 lime
- 1 tablespoon dark rum
- Sea salt
- 1 tablespoon vanilla extract

Method

Drain the tofu and blitz it in the food processor until smooth.

Melt the chocolate.

Add the chocolate and remaining ingredients into the food processor.

Mix until a mousse forms.

Refrigerate for at least 30 minutes before serving.

Apple and Peanut Butter Sarnies

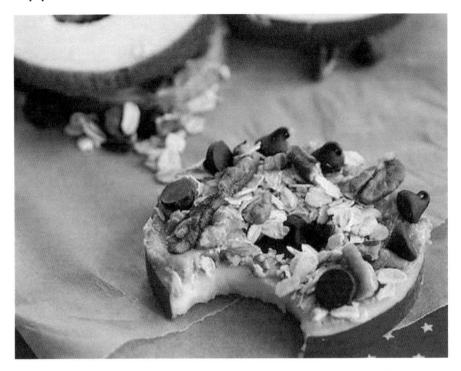

A sandwich for dessert you say? What's going on? This clever little recipe uses fresh apple slices as bread' and peanut butter, nuts, choc chips and sultanas as a sweet filling. Healthy and naughty – the perfect balance for a vegan dessert!

Ingredients

- Fresh apple (sliced into rings)
- Peanut butter (no added salt or sugar)
- Sultanas or raisins
- Ground nuts
- Dairy free chocolate chips (check out the baking aisle for dark choc chips)

- 1 tsp. cinnamon

Method

Core the apples and slice into rings (less than 1cm thick, for ease of cutting into).

Slather one slice of apple with peanut butter and top with raisins, choc chips and nuts.

Sprinkle cinnamon on the top and place another ring above to complete the sandwich.

Place on a baking tray lined with baking parchment and bake for 10 minutes at 350 degrees Fahrenheit.

Lemon and Berry Cheesecake

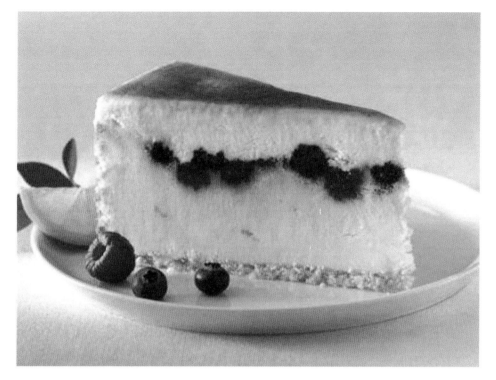

Another raw vegan dessert, this cheesecake is chock full of natural enzymes, a guilt-free and healthier adaptation of the traditional dairy dessert. Any assortment of berries can be used for this cheesecake, you could go for raspberries or blueberries, or even go all out and create a 'forest fruits' cheesecake using a range of different berries. The contrasting zest of the lemon and the sweetness of the berries make this dessert a truly indulging experience.

Ingredients

- 1 cup pitted dates

- 2 cups almonds (raw)
- ¾ cup lemon juice (freshly squeezed)
- 3 cups cashews (soaked for at least 60 minutes)
- ¾ cup agave nectar
- ¾ cup liquid coconut oil
- 1 teaspoon vanilla extract
- ½ cup water
- ½ teaspoon sea salt
- 3 cups frozen berries
- ½ cup dates or agave nectar (for berry sauce)

Method

Place almonds and dates into the food processor and blend to create the cheesecake base.

Press the mixture into the base of a spring form pan.

Blend the cashews, lemon juice, agave, coconut oil, water, vanilla extract and sea salt in the food processor to create the cream cheese.

Blend until smooth.

Pour cheese mixture onto the crust and tap the pan on the work surface to remove any air bubbles trapped in the mix.

Place cheesecake into the freezer for 3-4 hours, allowing firming to occur.

Transfer to fridge and remove when ready to eat (please note that coconut oil will melt at a warm temperature, so don't keep the cheesecake out of the fridge for long periods).

Make the berry sauce by blending the berries and dates (or agave) until smooth, slather on top of cake when serving and decorate the cake with a few whole berries.

.

Chocolate Oranges

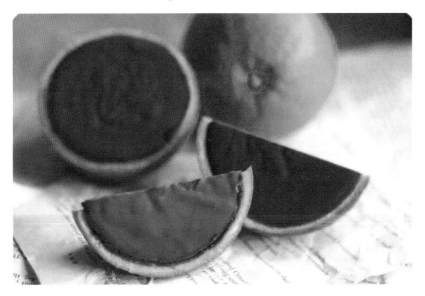

Ingredients

- 5 oranges, mandarins or clementines (peeled and separated)
- ½ cup dark chocolate pieces
- Sea salt

Method

Line a baking tray with parchment paper.

Place the chocolate pieces into a small glass bowl and place over boiling water in a saucepan, medium to low heat.

Once the chocolate has melted, take each orange slice and dip it halfway in the chocolate, place it onto the tray, then place into the fridge to harden the chocolate.

Place them into a serving bowl and enjoy!

Coconut Water Fruit Pops

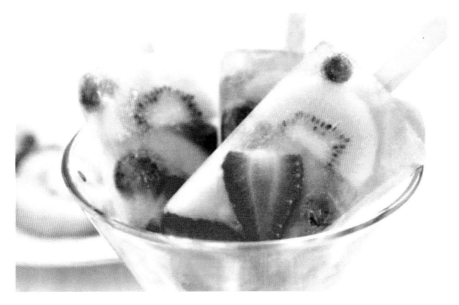

Ingredients

- 2 kiwis (halved and sliced)
- 8 strawberries (halved)
- 16 blueberries
- 16 raspberries
- 1 ½ cups coconut water
- Popsicle molds

Method

Fill the popsicle molds with an equal amount of the fruit.

Then fill with coconut water to the top.

Place the popsicle sticks on top of each, then place into the freezer and freeze for at least 5 hours or until solid.

Take them out of the freezer and enjoy!

Ambercup Coconut Milk Dessert

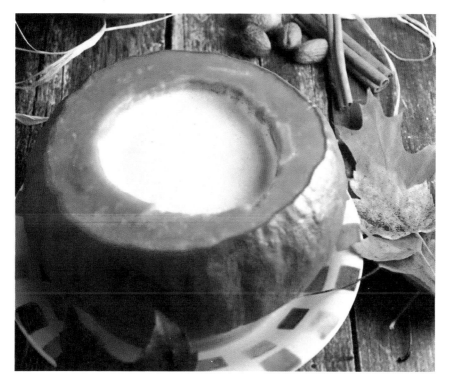

Ingredients

- 1 ambercup squash (Pumpkin substitute)
- 2 cups coconut milk
- ¼ cup agave nectar
- 2 tsp. ground cinnamon
- 1 chia egg white
- ¼ tsp nutmeg

Method

Start by cutting the top off of the squash and spoon out all of the seeds inside.

Place the squash into a large saucepan and add with a few inches of water, but not enough to cover the squash. Place onto a plate and set aside.

Simmer over a medium heat for about 15 minutes until the flesh inside is soft.

In a bowl, add the agave, coconut milk, chia egg white, cinnamon and nutmeg and stir to combine.

Pour the coconut mixture into the squash, use it as a bowl. Eat the squash as with the coconut mixture.

Serve and enjoy!

Baked Apple Chips

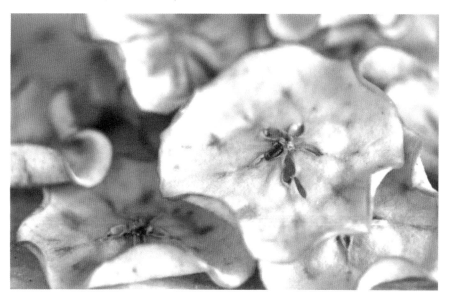

Ingredients

- 3 apples
- Ground cinnamon to taste

Method

Preheat oven to 220°F.

Line a baking tray with parchment paper and set aside.

Slice the apples thinly and place onto the baking tray. Dust some cinnamon on top of them and place them into the oven for 1 hour.

Then flip the slices and cook for another hour.

Take them out of the oven and allow them to cool.

Serve and enjoy this tasty little treat!

Creamed Spinach

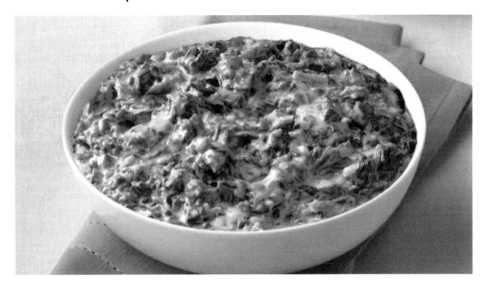

Ingredients

- 2 cups baby spinach
- 2 cups coconut milk
- 1 onion (finely chopped)
- 3 crushed garlic cloves
- 2 tbsp tapioca starch
- Pinch ground nutmeg
- Pinch cayenne pepper
- 3 tbsp sunflower seed butter
- Sea salt

Method

In a saucepan melt the ghee over a medium heat.

Then slowly whisk in the tapioca starch and cook for 5 mins.

Add the garlic and onion to the saucepan and cook for another minute.

Then add all of the spinach and cook until softened.

Add in the cayenne pepper, coconut milk and nutmeg, stir everything and cook for another 5 minutes.

Season with sea salt and serve.

Carrot and Rutabaga Mash

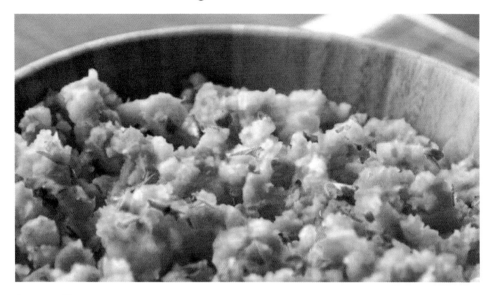

Ingredients

- 1 ¼ cup rutabaga (peeled and chopped)
- 1 ¼ cup carrots (peeled and chopped)
- 4 tbsp coconut oil
- 1 tbsp fresh parsley
- Sea salt
- Black pepper

Method

Place the rutabaga and carrots into a large saucepan and cover with water.

Bring the water to a boil on medium heat and reduce to a simmer. Then cover with a lid slightly and let it simmer for 20 minutes or until really soft.

Drain water and mash with a masher and add the coconut oil.

Season with the salt and pepper and sprinkle with fresh parsley to serve.

Berry Crumble

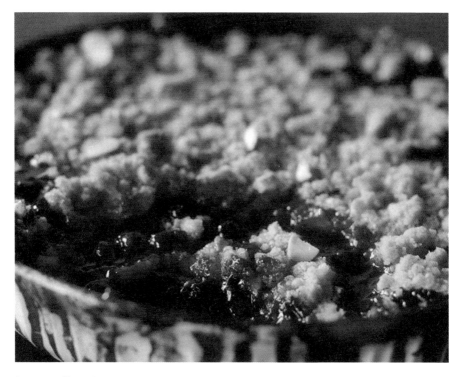

Ingredients

- 4 cups fresh or frozen mixed berries
- 1 cup almond meal
- ½ cup almond butter
- 1 cup oven roasted walnuts, sunflower seeds, pistachios.
- ½ tsp ground cinnamon

Method

Preheat oven to 350°F.

Crush the nuts using a mortar and pestle.

In a bowl, combine the nut mix, almond meal, cinnamon and ghee and combine well.

In a pie dish, spread half the nut mixture over the bottom of the dish, then top with the berries and finish with the rest of the nut mixture.

Bake for 30 minutes and serve warm with natural vanilla yogurt.

Marinated Beets

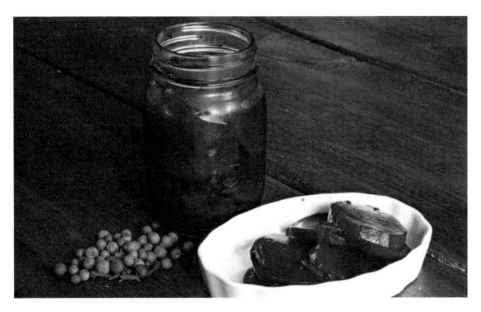

Ingredients

- 3 cups sliced beets
- 2 onions (sliced in thin rounds)
- 1 tbsp sunflower seed oil
- 2 sprigs fresh thyme
- 1 cup white wine vinegar
- ½ tsp sea salt
- 6 garlic cloves
- Pinch black pepper
- 2 x 1 quart jars

Method

Preheat oven to 400°F.

Prepare the beets by scrubbing them of any excess dirt and remove the root and stems.

Line a large baking dish with foil and place the beets onto there and drizzle with one tablespoon of sunflower oil.

Garnish them with thyme. Then seal the excess foil over the beets and roast for 1 to 1 ½ hours until soft.

Now, remove from the oven and allow to cool. When they are warm remove the skin, then allow to cool completely.

Place the onions into a large bowl and cover with hot water so that they begin to tender, for 10 minutes.

When the beets have cooled, slice them into ¼ inch rounds.

Once the 10 minutes has passed, start layering the onions and beets in the jars.

In a small mixing bowl, add the salt, cloves, pepper and vinegar, mix to combine. Then, pour half of the mixture into each jar.

Seal the jars then place them into the fridge for at least one day before serving.

Coffee Flavored Chocolate Mousse

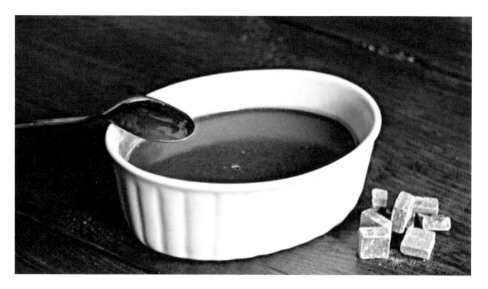

Ingredients

- ¼ cup dark chocolate chips or squares
- 1 tbsp. ground coffee beans
- 1 tbsp. vanilla extract
- ½ cup coconut milk
- ¼ cup boiling water
- 1/4 tsp mint extract

Method

In a medium skillet, melt the chocolate over a low heat to prevent burning and stir frequently with a wooden spoon.

Add in the coconut milk and combine with the chocolate.

In a small bowl, mix the boiling water with the ground coffee beans.

Now, combine the coffee bean mixture, chocolate mixture, vanilla and mint extract.

Pour the mixture into 2 large dessert dishes and place into the fridge for 2 - 3 hours. To allow them to become firm.

Take them out of the fridge and enjoy!

Maple Roasted Parsnip Chips

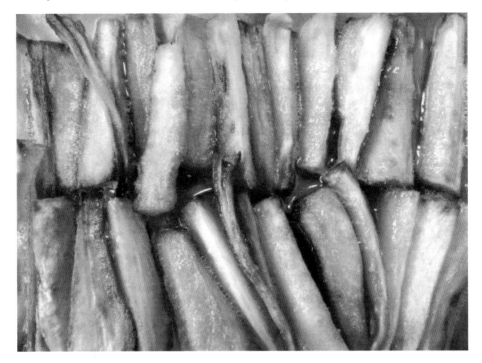

Ingredients

- 5 cups parsnips
- ¼ cup coconut oil
- 3 tbsp maple syrup

Method

Preheat oven to 392°F.

Peel the parsnips, cut them into chip sizes and place them into an oven proof dish.

Drizzle with coconut oil generously until covered and then do the same with the maple syrup.

Bake in the oven for 15 minutes, until crisp.

Remove from the oven and turn them over to cook on the other side for another 10 – 15 minutes.

Remove from oven, allow to cool and then serve.

Gingerbread Cookies

Ingredients

- 1 cup almonds
- ½ cup desiccated coconut
- ½ cup coconut milk
- 2 chia eggs
- 15 pitted dates
- 2 tbsp coconut oil
- 1 tsp allspice
- 1 tbsp cinnamon
- 1 tbsp ginger powder

Method

Preheat oven to 300°F.

If the dates are hard, soak them in coconut milk for 15 minutes.

Add the desiccated coconut and almonds into a food processor and process until they are finely ground. Then transfer to a bowl.

Now, process the dates, chia eggs, coconut milk, coconut oil and spices until smooth.

Stir the almond mixture into the coconut milk mixture and combine.

Line a baking tray with parchment paper and spread 2 tablespoons of the mixture onto it, like you would dough cookies, or you can use cookie cutters and add it to them.

Sprinkle the cookies with a bit more desiccated coconut and place into the oven for 15 minutes or until hard and golden brown.

Serve with a glass of almond milk.

Vinegar & Salt Kale Chips

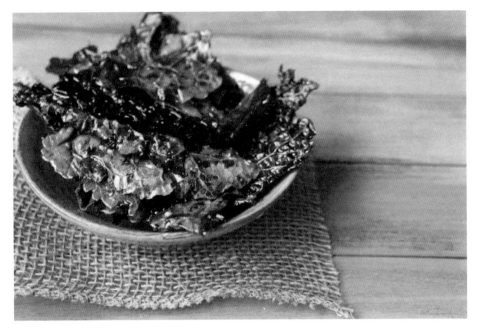

Ingredients

- 1 tsp. extra virgin olive oil
- 1 head kale, chopped
- 1 tbsp. apple cider vinegar
- ½ tsp. sea salt

Method

Place kale in a bowl and drizzle with vinegar and extra virgin olive oil; sprinkle with salt and massage the ingredients with hands.

Spread the kale out onto two paper-lined baking sheets and bake at 375°F for about 12 minutes or until crispy.

Let cool for about 10 minutes before serving.

Healthy Sautéed Kale

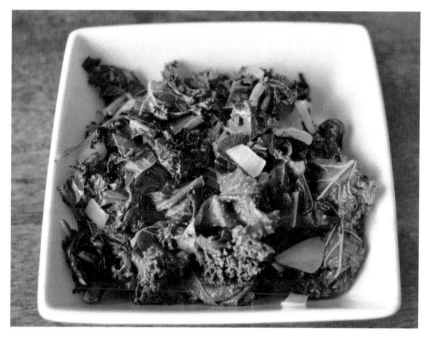

Ingredients

- 1 bunch kale, chopped
- 1 medium onion, chopped
- 2 tbsp. extra virgin olive oil
- ¼ tsp. sea salt

Method

Heat extra virgin olive oil in a pan set over medium heat. Stir in onion and sauté over medium low heat for about 15 minutes or until caramelized.

Stir in kale and sauté for 5 more minutes. Season with salt to serve.

Fig Tapenade

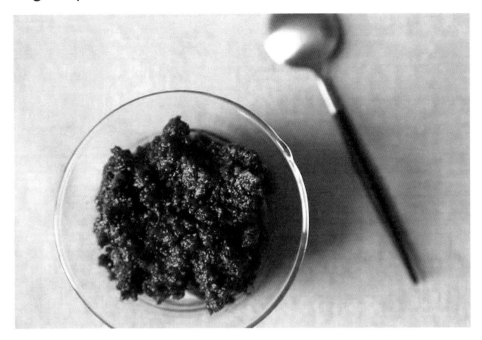

Ingredients

- 1 cup dried figs
- ½ tsp. apple cider vinegar
- 1 tbsp. extra virgin olive oil
- 1 cup kalamata olives
- 1 tbsp. chopped fresh thyme
- ½ cup water

Method

Pulse the figs in a food processor until well chopped; add water and continue pulsing to form a paste. Add olives and pulse until well blended.

Add thyme, vinegar and extra virgin olive oil and pulse until very smooth. Serve with chestnut crackers.

Carrot French Fries

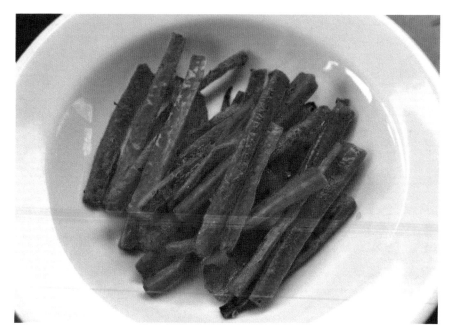

Ingredients

- 2 tbsp. extra virgin olive oil
- 6 large carrots
- ½ tsp. sea salt

Method

Chop the carrots into 2-inch sections and then cut each section into thin sticks.

Toss together the carrots sticks with extra virgin olive oil and salt in a bowl and spread into a baking sheet lined with parchment paper.

Bake the carrot sticks at 425° for about 20 minutes or until

Made in the USA
Columbia, SC
24 May 2018